LOW POTASSIUM DIET FOR WOMEN

The complete guide with homemade recipes to manage Hyperkalemia for women.

Berlinda Harrison

TABLE OF CONTENTS

INTRODUCTION

Embarking on the journey of a low potassium diet, especially for women, is akin to navigating a river that twists and turns through the landscape of nutrition and health. It's a path that requires a map, a compass, and a good sense of humor, especially when you find yourself eyeing a banana with suspicion, wondering, "Is this yellow delight friend or foe today?"

Why, you might ask, should this particular dietary path demand your attention amidst the cacophony of dietary advice bombarding us from all sides? The answer lies not just in the unique role potassium plays in our bodies but also in the nuanced needs of women's health—a topic that, much like the last cookie in the jar, often feels just out of reach.

Potassium, that enigmatic mineral, is a bit like the unsung hero of a blockbuster movie. It's always there, performing crucial tasks behind the scenes—regulating heart rhythms, ensuring muscle function, and maintaining fluid balance, to name a few. Yet, it rarely gets the spotlight until something goes awry. Too much or too little can lead to a plot twist in our body's finely tuned operations, with women often facing unique challenges in maintaining this delicate balance.

This book, "Low Potassium Diet for Women," is your invitation to a grand adventure, one that promises not just to alter your dietary habits but to transform your understanding of how nutrition shapes your health and well-being. It's written for you—the curious, the health-conscious, the seekers of balance and wellness in a world that often seems to spin too fast on its axis.

Why focus on women, you might wonder? Well, it's not just because we're fabulous (which we are, by the way). It's because our bodies are masterpieces of complexity, influenced by hormones, reproductive health, and life stages from the whirlwind of adolescence to the wisdom of menopause. These factors can affect how our bodies process minerals, including potassium. This book aims to peel back the layers of dietary advice to reveal the core information you need to navigate your health journey with confidence.

As we dive into the world of low potassium diets, we'll explore the shores of scientific research and sail through practical advice, all while keeping the journey light-hearted. After all, who said dietary changes have to be as dreary as a rainy day without an umbrella? We'll share laughs over the perplexities of portion sizes, the mysteries of meal planning, and the occasional culinary misadventure (because who hasn't had one of those?).

But this book is more than just a collection of facts and guidelines. It's a companion for your journey, one that understands the challenges of making dietary changes and the triumphs that come with discovering delicious, healthful foods that support your well-being. It's here to offer a hand to hold (figuratively speaking, of course) as you make choices that nourish not just your body but your spirit.

You might be thinking, "But why a low potassium diet? Can't I just eat what I've always eaten and be fine?" It's a fair question. For some, the path of least resistance is indeed the path of choice. However, for those who find themselves grappling with health conditions that necessitate a closer look at potassium intake—be it kidney issues, concerns about heart health, or the desire to fine-tune one's diet for optimal wellness—this book is a beacon, illuminating the way forward.

We'll explore the signs that might indicate a need to adjust your potassium intake, from the whispers of fatigue to the more assertive nudges of muscle cramps or changes in heart rhythm. Understanding these signals is the first step in becoming an advocate for your health, a theme that weaves through the pages of this book like a golden thread.

But fear not; this journey is not about restriction or deprivation. On the contrary, it's about discovery and delight in the abundance of foods that can nourish and satisfy. It's about learning to listen to your body's needs and responding with love and care. And yes, it's also about finding joy in the kitchen, experimenting with flavors and textures, and perhaps even surprising yourself with a newfound love for cooking.

As we embark on this adventure together, remember that every journey begins with a single step—or in this case, a single page turn. With each chapter, you'll gain insights and tools to help you navigate the low potassium diet with ease and confidence. You'll learn not just what to eat but how to think about food in a way that supports your health goals and lifestyle.

WHY A LOW POTASSIUM DIET IS NECESSARY FOR WOMEN

In the realm of nutrition and health, the significance of dietary potassium cannot be overstated, particularly for women. Potassium, a vital mineral, plays a crucial role in maintaining several bodily functions, including fluid balance, nerve signals, and muscle contractions. However, while the importance of potassium is widely recognized, less attention is often given to the circumstances under which a low potassium diet might be necessary, especially for women. As a professional nutritionist, it's imperative to explore the nuanced needs of women's health and why, in specific instances, a reduction in potassium intake is not only beneficial but necessary.

Women's bodies undergo various physiological changes throughout their lives, such as menstruation, pregnancy, and menopause, each presenting unique nutritional demands. These changes can affect how the body processes and requires nutrients, including potassium. For instance, certain health conditions that disproportionately affect women, such as kidney disorders, hypertension, and osteoporosis, can necessitate a careful examination of potassium intake.

Kidney disorders, which can impair the body's ability to regulate potassium levels, are of particular concern. High potassium levels, or hyperkalemia, can lead to serious health issues, including heart rhythm problems, which could be fatal. Women with chronic kidney disease or those on certain medications that affect kidney function may need to adopt a low potassium diet to manage their condition effectively and prevent complications.

Moreover, hypertension, a condition that affects a significant portion of the adult population, has been linked to dietary potassium intake. While potassium can help lower blood pressure by balancing out the negative effects of salt, in individuals with kidney issues or those who cannot excrete potassium efficiently, a lower potassium intake is advised to avoid exacerbating high blood pressure and related cardiovascular risks.

Osteoporosis, another condition with a high prevalence among women, especially post-menopausal women, highlights the complex relationship between potassium and bone health. Some studies suggest that a diet high in fruits and vegetables, which are potassium-rich, can improve bone density. However, for women with conditions affecting potassium excretion, the focus shifts towards balancing potassium intake to support bone health without risking hyperkalemia.

It's crucial to approach the concept of a low potassium diet with a personalized perspective, recognizing that the dietary needs of women can vary widely based on individual health status, age, and lifestyle factors. A professional nutritionist understands that dietary advice must be tailored to the individual, taking into account the whole picture of a person's health, including their risk factors for diseases that may be impacted by potassium levels.

In advising a low potassium diet, the goal is not to eliminate potassium from the diet—such an approach would be neither feasible nor healthy, given potassium's essential roles in the body. Instead, the aim is to moderate intake, focusing on foods that provide the necessary nutrients without exceeding the recommended potassium levels for those who need to limit their intake. This involves a careful selection of fruits, vegetables, grains, and proteins, guided by a thorough understanding of how different foods contribute to overall potassium levels.

GETTING STARTED

When it comes to controlling your potassium intake, knowing where you are and where you need to go is the first step. This chapter is meant to be your guide, your map, and your traveling partner as you set out on this journey. Starting a journey toward a healthier you can often feel like you are standing at the base of a mountain, looking up. It's both thrilling and daunting.

Assessing Your Potassium Intake

Understanding your current potassium intake is akin to taking stock of what's in your backpack before a hike. You need to know what you have to ensure you're not carrying too much weight—in this case, potassium.

Start by keeping a food diary for a week. Write down everything you eat and drink, no matter how small. There are several apps and tools available that can help you track your food intake and automatically calculate your daily potassium intake. This exercise is eye-opening for many, as it reveals not just your potassium intake but also your dietary habits.

Next, compare your average daily intake to the recommended dietary allowance (RDA) for potassium. For most women, the RDA is around 2,600 to 2,800 mg per day. However, if you're on a low potassium diet, your doctor might recommend a lower intake. This comparison will give you a clear picture of where adjustments need to be made.

Remember, potassium is found in many foods, not just bananas. It's abundant in fruits, vegetables, dairy products, and meats. Learning to identify high-potassium foods and understanding how to balance your diet will be crucial. But don't worry, this isn't about deprivation. It's about making informed choices that support your health goals.

Setting Goals for a Low Potassium Diet

Setting goals is like plotting waypoints on your journey. They give you direction and help measure your progress. When it comes to adjusting your diet, specificity is your friend. Instead of a vague "eat less potassium," set clear, achievable goals. For example, "reduce my daily potassium intake to 2,000 mg per day."

Work with a nutritionist to create a meal plan that meets your nutritional needs while staying within your potassium limits. This plan should include a variety of foods to ensure you're getting a balanced diet. Remember, the goal is to reduce potassium, not eliminate it entirely, as it's still a vital nutrient for your body.

Setting smaller, weekly goals can also help make the transition easier. For instance, you could start by replacing one high-potassium food in your diet with a lower-potassium alternative each week. Celebrate these small victories; they add up to significant changes over time.

Understanding Potassium's Role in Women's Health

Potassium plays several critical roles in the body. It helps regulate heart function, muscle contractions, and fluid balance. For women, the importance of potassium is magnified by the unique aspects of women's health, such as hormonal fluctuations and the demands of pregnancy and breastfeeding.

However, too much potassium can lead to hyperkalemia, a condition that can cause heart palpitations, muscle weakness, and other serious health issues. Women with kidney issues or those taking certain medications may be at higher risk and need to monitor their potassium intake more closely.

Understanding these risks and how potassium interacts with your body can empower you to make informed decisions about your diet. It's not just about following a list of "do's and don'ts." It's about understanding why those recommendations exist and how they benefit you.

BASICS OF A LOW POTASSIUM DIET

A comprehensive grasp of nutrition, an attention to detail, and a dedication to making well-informed food decisions are necessary before committing to a low-potassium diet. This chapter aims to give you the information and resources you need to properly follow this nutritional plan..

Identifying High Potassium Foods

Understanding which foods are high in potassium is the cornerstone of managing a low potassium diet. Potassium is a mineral essential for the body's normal functioning, playing a key role in heart health, muscle function, and nerve transmission. However, for individuals with certain health conditions, such as kidney disease, or those on specific medications, managing potassium intake is crucial to avoid the risk of hyperkalemia—a condition characterized by too much potassium in the blood, which can lead to serious health complications.

High potassium foods include:

- Fruits such as bananas, oranges, avocados, and melons.

- Vegetables like potatoes, tomatoes, spinach, and broccoli.

- Dairy products, particularly milk and yogurt.

- Whole grains and nuts.

- Beans and legumes.

To effectively identify high potassium foods, it's essential to become familiar with nutritional content resources, such as databases and food labels, which provide detailed information on the potassium content of various foods. Additionally, consulting with a nutritionist or dietitian can offer personalized guidance based on your specific health needs and dietary restrictions.

When planning your diet, consider the portion size, as it significantly affects the total intake of potassium. Opting for smaller portions of high potassium foods can help manage your overall potassium levels without completely eliminating these nutrient-rich foods from your diet.

Tips for Reading Food Labels

Reading food labels is a skill that becomes invaluable when managing a low potassium diet. Food labels provide critical information about the nutritional content of packaged foods, including their potassium content. However, not all food labels include potassium, so it's important to know which nutrients can indicate the presence of potassium.

Here are some tips for effectively reading food labels:

1. **Check the Serving Size**: The nutritional information is based on the serving size listed on the package. Comparing this to the amount you actually consume is crucial for accurately assessing your intake.

2. **Look for Potassium Content**: If potassium is listed, it will be found in the mineral section of the nutrition facts. The amount is usually given in milligrams (mg).

3. **Understand Daily Value Percentages**: The % Daily Value (%DV) helps you understand how much a nutrient in a serving of food contributes to a daily diet. For potassium, the goal is to stay below a certain %DV, based on your healthcare provider's recommendations.

4. **Identify Ingredients High in Potassium**: Even if potassium isn't listed, ingredients like potassium chloride, a common salt substitute, indicate high potassium content. Learning to recognize these ingredients can help you make better choices.

Developing the habit of reading food labels can empower you to make informed decisions about the foods you include in your diet, ensuring you stay within your potassium limits while still enjoying a varied and nutritious diet.

Planning Balanced Low Potassium Meals

Planning balanced low potassium meals is both an art and a science. It involves understanding the nutritional content of foods, creatively combining ingredients to meet dietary needs, and ensuring meals are satisfying and enjoyable.

Start by focusing on low potassium foods that can form the basis of your meals:

- Fruits: Apples, berries, and peaches.

- Vegetables: Cabbage, carrots, and green beans.

- Protein: Lean meats, poultry, and fish. Consider portion sizes to manage protein intake, as some sources can be higher in potassium.

- Grains: Rice, pasta, and bread are generally low in potassium, but whole grains can have more, so moderation is key.

When planning meals, aim for variety to ensure you're getting a broad spectrum of nutrients. Incorporate different colors of fruits and vegetables to benefit from a range of vitamins and minerals. Use herbs and spices to add flavor without increasing potassium content.

Meal planning tips:

1. **Create a Weekly Menu**: Planning ahead can help you balance your meals and make grocery shopping more efficient.

2. **Cook in Batches**: Preparing meals in advance can save time and ensure you have low potassium options readily available.

3. **Adjust Recipes**: Modify your favorite recipes to lower their potassium content by substituting high potassium ingredients with lower potassium alternatives.

Remember, managing a low potassium diet doesn't mean sacrificing flavor or enjoyment. With careful planning and a bit of creativity, you can enjoy delicious, balanced meals that support your health goals.

BREAKFAST RECIPES

Apple Cinnamon Oatmeal

Prep Time: 5 mins

Cook Time: 10 mins

Total Time: 15 mins

Servings: 2

Yield: 2 servings

Ingredients:

- 1 cup rolled oats
- 2 cups water
- 1 medium apple, peeled and diced
- 1/2 teaspoon cinnamon
- 1 tablespoon honey
- 1/4 cup almond milk
- A pinch of salt

Directions:

1. In a medium saucepan, bring the water to a boil. Add the oats and a pinch of salt, then reduce the heat to medium-low.

2. Stir in the diced apple and cinnamon. Cook for about 5 minutes, or until the oats are soft and the water is mostly absorbed.

3. Remove from heat and stir in the honey and almond milk, adjusting the sweetness and creaminess to your liking.

4. Serve warm, with an extra sprinkle of cinnamon on top for garnish.

Nutrition Facts (per serving)

- Calories: 190
- Fat: 2.5g
- Carbohydrates: 36g
- Protein: 5g

Veggie Egg Muffins

Prep Time: 10 mins

Cook Time: 20 mins

Total Time: 30 mins

Servings: 6

Yield: 12 muffins

Ingredients:

- 8 large eggs
- 1/4 cup milk
- 1/2 cup diced tomatoes
- 1/2 cup diced zucchini
- 1/2 cup shredded cheddar cheese
- Salt and pepper to taste

Directions:

1. Preheat the oven to 350°F (175°C) and grease a 12-cup muffin tin.

2. In a large bowl, whisk together the eggs and milk. Season with salt and pepper.

3. Stir in the diced tomatoes, zucchini, and shredded cheese.

4. Pour the egg mixture evenly into the muffin cups.

5. Bake for 20 minutes, or until the egg muffins are set and lightly golden on top.

6. Let them cool for a few minutes before removing from the tin. Serve warm.

Nutrition Facts (per serving)

- Calories: 140

- Fat: 9g

- Carbohydrates: 2g

- Protein: 12g

Berry Smoothie Bowl

Prep Time: 5 mins

Cook Time: 0 mins

Total Time: 5 mins

Servings: 1

Yield: 1 serving

Ingredients:

- 1 cup frozen mixed berries

- 1/2 banana, 1/4 cup Greek yogurt

- 1/2 cup almond milk

- Toppings: sliced almonds, chia seeds, fresh berries

Directions:

1. In a blender, combine the frozen berries, banana, Greek yogurt, and almond milk. Blend until smooth.

2. Pour the smoothie into a bowl and garnish with your choice of toppings, such as sliced almonds, chia seeds, and fresh berries.

Nutrition Facts (per serving)

- Calories: 220

- Fat: 4g

- Carbohydrates: 40g

- Protein: 10g

Avocado Toast with Egg

Prep Time: 5 mins, Cook Time: 5 mins

Total Time: 10 mins

Servings: 1

Yield: 1 serving

Ingredients:

- 1 slice whole grain bread

- 1/2 ripe avocado

- 1 egg, cooked to your liking (poached, fried, or scrambled)

- Salt and pepper to taste

- Red pepper flakes (optional)

Directions:

1. Toast the bread to your liking,

2. Mash the avocado and spread it evenly on the toast.

3. Top with the cooked egg. Season with salt, pepper, and red pepper flakes if desired.

Nutrition Facts (per serving)

- Calories: 300

- Fat: 20g

- Carbohydrates: 20g

- Protein: 13g

Greek Yogurt Parfait

Prep Time: 5 mins, Cook Time: 0 mins

Total Time: 5 mins

Servings: 1

Yield: 1 serving

Ingredients:

- 1 cup Greek yogurt

- 1/4 cup granola

- 1/2 cup fresh strawberries, sliced

- 1 tablespoon honey

Directions:

1. In a serving glass or bowl, layer half of the Greek yogurt.

2. Add a layer of granola, then a layer of sliced strawberries.

3. Repeat the layers with the remaining ingredients.

4. Drizzle honey over the top before serving.

Nutrition Facts (per serving)

- Calories: 320

- Fat: 6g

- Carbohydrates: 46g

- Protein: 20g

Spinach and Feta Omelette

Prep Time: 5 mins

Cook Time: 10 mins

Total Time: 15 mins

Servings: 1

Yield: 1 omelette

Ingredients:

- 2 large eggs
- 1 tablespoon water
- 1/2 cup fresh spinach, chopped
- 1/4 cup feta cheese, crumbled
- Salt and pepper to taste
- 1 teaspoon olive oil

Directions:

1. In a bowl, whisk together the eggs, water, salt, and pepper.
2. Heat olive oil in a non-stick skillet over medium heat. Add the spinach and sauté until wilted, about 2 minutes.
3. Pour the egg mixture over the spinach. Cook for a few minutes until the edges start to set.
4. Sprinkle feta cheese over half of the omelette. Fold the other half over the cheese and continue cooking until the cheese is slightly melted and the eggs are cooked to your liking.
5. Serve immediately, seasoned with additional salt and pepper if desired.

Nutrition Facts (per serving)

- Calories: 250

- Fat: 18g

- Carbohydrates: 2g

- Protein: 20g

Peanut Butter and Banana Sandwich

Prep Time: 5 mins, Cook Time: 0 mins

Total Time: 5 mins

Servings: 1

Yield: 1 sandwich

Ingredients:

- 2 slices whole grain bread

- 2 tablespoons peanut butter

- 1/2 banana, thinly sliced

- A sprinkle of cinnamon (optional)

Directions:

1. Spread peanut butter evenly on one slice of bread.

2. Arrange banana slices over the peanut butter. Sprinkle with cinnamon if using.

3. Top with the second slice of bread. Press down gently.

4. Cut the sandwich in half and serve.

Nutrition Facts (per serving)

- Calories: 330

- Fat: 16g

- Carbohydrates: 40g

- Protein: 12g

Cottage Cheese with Pineapple

Prep Time: 5 mins

Cook Time: 0 mins

Total Time: 5 mins

Servings: 1

Yield: 1 serving

Ingredients:

- 1/2 cup low-fat cottage cheese
- 1/2 cup pineapple chunks, fresh or canned in juice (drained)
- 1 teaspoon honey (optional)

Directions:

1. In a bowl, combine the cottage cheese and pineapple chunks.
2. Drizzle with honey if desired.
3. Mix gently and serve chilled.

Nutrition Facts (per serving)

- Calories: 180
- Fat: 2g
- Carbohydrates: 25g
- Protein: 15g

Turkey and Avocado Wrap

Prep Time: 10 mins

Cook Time: 0 mins

Total Time: 10 mins

Servings: 1

Yield: 1 wrap

Ingredients:

- 1 whole grain tortilla
- 2 slices turkey breast
- 1/4 avocado, thinly sliced
- 1/4 cup lettuce, shredded
- 1 tablespoon ranch dressing
- Salt and pepper to taste

Directions:

1. Lay the tortilla flat on a plate.
2. Arrange turkey slices, avocado slices, and shredded lettuce over the tortilla.
3. Drizzle with ranch dressing and season with salt and pepper.
4. Roll the tortilla tightly, cut in half, and serve.

Nutrition Facts (per serving)

- Calories: 320
- Fat: 15g
- Carbohydrates: 28g
- Protein: 20g

Blueberry Almond Overnight Oats

Prep Time: 5 mins

Cook Time: 0 mins (Refrigerate overnight)

Total Time: 8 hrs 5 mins

Servings: 1

Yield: 1 serving

Ingredients:

- 1/2 cup rolled oats
- 1/2 cup almond milk
- 1/4 cup blueberries
- 1 tablespoon sliced almonds
- 1 tablespoon chia seeds
- 1 teaspoon honey or maple syrup

Directions:

1. In a mason jar or airtight container, combine the rolled oats, almond milk, blueberries, sliced almonds, and chia seeds.
2. Sweeten with honey or maple syrup, and stir well to combine.
3. Seal the container and refrigerate overnight, allowing the oats to soften and the flavors to meld.
4. In the morning, stir the oats well. If the mixture is too thick, add a little more almond milk to reach your desired consistency.
5. Serve cold or at room temperature.

Nutrition Facts (per serving)

- Calories: 300
- Fat: 10g
- Carbohydrates: 45g
- Protein: 10g

LUNCH

Chicken Caesar Salad Wrap

Prep Time: 10 mins

Cook Time: 0 mins

Total Time: 10 mins

Servings: 2

Yield: 2 wrap

Ingredients:

- 2 whole grain tortillas
- 1 cup cooked chicken breast, sliced
- 1 cup romaine lettuce, chopped
- 1/4 cup Caesar dressing, low sodium
- 2 tablespoons grated Parmesan cheese
- Black pepper to taste

Directions:

1. Lay the tortillas flat on a clean surface.
2. Divide the chicken slices evenly among the tortillas, placing them in the center.
3. Top the chicken with chopped romaine lettuce.
4. Drizzle Caesar dressing over the lettuce and sprinkle with Parmesan cheese. Add black pepper to taste.
5. Carefully fold the sides of the tortilla in, then roll up tightly to enclose the filling.
6. Cut each wrap in half and serve immediately for a refreshing and satisfying lunch.

Nutrition Facts (per serving)

- Calories: 350
- Fat: 15g
- Carbohydrates: 27g
- Protein: 25g

Turkey and Avocado Salad

Prep Time: 15 mins

Cook Time: 0 mins

Total Time: 15 mins

Servings: 4

Yield: 4 servings

Ingredients:

- 2 cups cooked turkey breast, diced
- 1 ripe avocado, diced
- 1/2 cup cherry tomatoes, halved
- 1/4 cup red onion, finely chopped
- 2 tablespoons olive oil
- 1 tablespoon lemon juice
- Salt and pepper to taste
- 4 cups mixed salad greens

Directions:

1. In a large bowl, combine the diced turkey, avocado, cherry tomatoes, and red onion.

2. In a small bowl, whisk together the olive oil and lemon juice. Season with salt and pepper.

3. Pour the dressing over the turkey mixture and toss gently to coat.

4. Serve the turkey and avocado mixture over a bed of mixed salad greens.

Nutrition Facts (per serving)

- Calories: 290

- Fat: 17g

- Carbohydrates: 8g

- Protein: 27g

Quinoa Vegetable Soup

Prep Time: 10 mins

Cook Time: 30 mins

Total Time: 40 mins

Servings: 6

Yield: 6 servings

Ingredients:

- 1 tablespoon olive oil

- 1/2 cup onion, chopped

- 2 garlic cloves, minced

- 1 carrot, diced

- 1 celery stalk, diced

- 1/2 cup quinoa, rinsed

- 4 cups vegetable broth, low sodium

- 1 cup diced tomatoes, canned with juice

- 1 teaspoon dried thyme

- 1 bay leaf

- Salt and pepper to taste

- 2 cups spinach leaves

Directions:

1. Heat olive oil in a large pot over medium heat. Add onion and garlic, sautéing until softened, about 5 minutes.

2. Add carrot and celery to the pot, cooking for another 5 minutes.

3. Stir in quinoa, vegetable broth, diced tomatoes, thyme, and bay leaf. Season with salt and pepper.

4. Bring to a boil, then reduce heat and simmer, covered, for 20 minutes or until quinoa is cooked.

5. Add spinach leaves and cook until wilted, about 2 minutes.

6. Remove the bay leaf before serving. Serve hot.

Nutrition Facts (per serving)

- Calories: 150

- Fat: 4g

- Carbohydrates: 23g

- Protein: 6g

Grilled Chicken and Vegetable Kabobs

Prep Time: 20 mins (plus marinating time)

Cook Time: 10 mins

Total Time: 30 mins

Servings: 4

Yield: 8 kabobs

Ingredients:

- 1 pound chicken breast, cut into 1-inch pieces
- 1 zucchini, sliced into rounds
- 1 bell pepper, cut into 1-inch pieces
- 1/2 red onion, cut into wedges
- 2 tablespoons olive oil
- 2 tablespoons lemon juice
- 1 teaspoon dried oregano
- Salt and pepper to taste

Directions:

1. In a bowl, whisk together olive oil, lemon juice, oregano, salt, and pepper. Add chicken pieces and toss to coat. Marinate for at least 30 minutes in the refrigerator.

2. Preheat grill to medium-high heat. Thread chicken, zucchini, bell pepper, and onion onto skewers.

3. Grill kabobs, turning occasionally, until chicken is cooked through and vegetables are tender, about 10 minutes.

4. Serve kabobs with a side of mixed greens or your choice of side salad.

Nutrition Facts (per serving)

- Calories: 250
- Fat: 9g
- Carbohydrates: 8g
- Protein: 34g

Tuna Salad Stuffed Avocado

Prep Time: 10 mins

Cook Time: 0 mins

Total Time: 10 mins

Servings: 2

Yield: 2 servings

Ingredients:

- 1 can (5 ounces) tuna in water, drained
- 2 tablespoons mayonnaise, low fat
- 1/4 cup cucumber, diced
- 1 tablespoon red onion, minced
- 1 teaspoon lemon juice
- Salt and pepper to taste
- 1 ripe avocado, halved and pitted

Directions:

1. In a bowl, mix together the tuna, mayonnaise, cucumber, red onion, and lemon juice. Season with salt and pepper to taste.

2. Scoop out some of the avocado flesh to create more space for the filling, leaving a thick border.

3. Divide the tuna salad evenly among the avocado halves.

4. Serve immediately, garnished with additional lemon juice or fresh herbs if desired.

Nutrition Facts (per serving)

- Calories: 290
- Fat: 21g

- Carbohydrates: 9g

- Protein: 19g

Chicken and Rice Soup

Prep Time: 10 mins

Cook Time: 30 mins

Total Time: 40 mins

Servings: 4

Yield: 4 servings

Ingredients:

- 1 tablespoon olive oil

- 1/2 cup carrots, diced

- 1/2 cup celery, diced

- 1/2 cup onion, diced

- 2 garlic cloves, minced

- 6 cups low-sodium chicken broth

- 1 cup cooked chicken breast, shredded

- 1/2 cup white rice

- 1 teaspoon dried thyme

- Salt and pepper to taste

- 2 tablespoons fresh parsley, chopped

Directions:

1. Heat olive oil in a large pot over medium heat. Add carrots, celery, onion, and garlic; sauté until vegetables are softened, about 5 minutes.

2. Pour in the chicken broth and bring to a boil. Add the shredded chicken, rice, and thyme. Season with salt and pepper.

3. Reduce heat to a simmer and cook, covered, until the rice is tender, about 20 minutes.

4. Stir in fresh parsley before serving. Serve hot.

Nutrition Facts (per serving)

- Calories: 220

- Fat: 5g

- Carbohydrates: 22g

- Protein: 20g

Beef and Broccoli Stir-Fry

Prep Time: 15 mins

Cook Time: 10 mins

Total Time: 25 mins

Servings: 4

Yield: 4 servings

Ingredients:

- 1 pound lean beef, thinly sliced

- 2 cups broccoli florets

- 1 tablespoon olive oil

- 2 garlic cloves, minced

- 1/4 cup low-sodium soy sauce

- 1 tablespoon cornstarch

- 1/2 cup water

- 1 teaspoon sesame oil

- Salt and pepper to taste

Directions:

1. In a small bowl, whisk together the soy sauce, cornstarch, water, and sesame oil. Set aside.

2. Heat olive oil in a large skillet or wok over medium-high heat. Add garlic and sauté for 30 seconds.

3. Add the beef and cook until browned, about 3-4 minutes. Remove beef from the skillet and set aside.

4. In the same skillet, add broccoli florets and a splash of water. Cover and cook until broccoli is tender, about 3 minutes.

5. Return the beef to the skillet. Pour the soy sauce mixture over the beef and broccoli. Cook, stirring constantly, until the sauce has thickened, about 2 minutes.

6. Season with salt and pepper to taste. Serve immediately.

Nutrition Facts (per serving)

- Calories: 250

- Fat: 10g

- Carbohydrates: 10g

- Protein: 30g

Spinach and Cheese Stuffed Chicken

Prep Time: 20 mins

Cook Time: 25 mins

Total Time: 45 mins

Servings: 4

Yield: 4 servings

Ingredients:

- 4 boneless, skinless chicken breasts
- 1 cup fresh spinach, chopped
- 1/2 cup ricotta cheese
- 1/4 cup grated Parmesan cheese
- Salt and pepper to taste
- 1 tablespoon olive oil

Directions:

1. Preheat oven to 375°F (190°C).

2. In a bowl, mix together the spinach, ricotta, and Parmesan cheese. Season with salt and pepper.

3. Cut a pocket into the side of each chicken breast. Stuff each with the spinach and cheese mixture. Secure with toothpicks if necessary.

4. Season the outside of the chicken with salt and pepper. Heat olive oil in a skillet over medium-high heat. Sear chicken on both sides until golden, about 3 minutes per side.

5. Transfer chicken to a baking dish and bake in the preheated oven until cooked through, about 20 minutes.

6. Serve hot, removing toothpicks before serving.

Nutrition Facts (per serving)

- Calories: 290
- Fat: 12g
- Carbohydrates: 2g
- Protein: 40g

Shrimp and Asparagus Salad

Prep Time: 15 mins

Cook Time: 5 mins

Total Time: 20 mins

Servings: 4

Yield: 4 servings

Ingredients:

- 1 pound shrimp, peeled and deveined
- 2 cups asparagus, trimmed and cut into 1-inch pieces
- 1 tablespoon olive oil
- Salt and pepper to taste
- 4 cups mixed salad greens
- 1/4 cup balsamic vinaigrette

Directions:

1. Heat olive oil in a skillet over medium-high heat. Add shrimp and asparagus. Season with salt and pepper. Cook, stirring occasionally, until shrimp are pink and opaque, about 4-5 minutes.

2. Arrange mixed salad greens on plates. Top with the cooked shrimp and asparagus.

3. Drizzle with balsamic vinaigrette before serving.

Nutrition Facts (per serving)

- Calories: 220
- Fat: 8g
- Carbohydrates: 8g
- Protein: 30g

Mediterranean Quinoa Salad

Prep Time: 15 mins

Cook Time: 15 mins

Total Time: 30 mins

Servings: 4

Yield: 4 servings

Ingredients:

- 1 cup quinoa, rinsed

- 2 cups water

- 1 cup cherry tomatoes, halved

- 1 cucumber, diced

- 1/2 cup Kalamata olives, pitted and halved

- 1/4 cup feta cheese, crumbled

- 1/4 cup red onion, finely chopped

- 2 tablespoons olive oil

- 1 tablespoon lemon juice

- Salt and pepper to taste

- 1 teaspoon dried oregano

Directions:

1. In a medium saucepan, bring water to a boil. Add quinoa and reduce heat to low. Cover and simmer until water is absorbed and quinoa is tender, about 15 minutes. Let cool.

2. In a large bowl, combine cooled quinoa, cherry tomatoes, cucumber, olives, feta cheese, and red onion.

3. In a small bowl, whisk together olive oil, lemon juice, salt, pepper, and oregano. Pour over the quinoa mixture and toss to combine.

4. Serve chilled or at room temperature.

Nutrition Facts (per serving)

- Calories: 280

- Fat: 14g

- Carbohydrates: 32g

- Protein: 8g

DINNER

Lemon Herb Baked Cod

Prep Time: 10 mins

Cook Time: 20 mins

Total Time: 30 mins

Servings: 4

Yield: 4 servings

Ingredients:

- 4 cod fillets
- 2 tablespoons olive oil
- 1 lemon, juiced and zested
- 2 garlic cloves, minced
- 1 teaspoon dried oregano
- 1 teaspoon dried thyme
- Salt and pepper to taste

Directions:

1. Preheat the oven to 400°F (200°C) and lightly grease a baking dish.

2. In a small bowl, mix together olive oil, lemon juice and zest, garlic, oregano, thyme, salt, and pepper.

3. Place cod fillets in the prepared baking dish and pour the lemon herb mixture over them, ensuring each fillet is evenly coated.

4. Bake in the preheated oven for 20 minutes, or until the fish flakes easily with a fork.

5. Serve immediately, garnished with additional lemon slices if desired.

Nutrition Facts (per serving)

- Calories: 200

- Fat: 10g

- Carbohydrates: 2g

- Protein: 25g

Stuffed Bell Peppers

Prep Time: 15 mins

Cook Time: 30 mins

Total Time: 45 mins

Servings: 4

Yield: 4 servings

Ingredients:

- 4 bell peppers, tops removed and seeded

- 1 pound ground turkey

- 1/2 cup onion, diced

- 1 cup cooked quinoa

- 1 cup spinach, chopped

- 1/2 cup tomato sauce, low sodium

- 1 teaspoon garlic powder

- 1 teaspoon smoked paprika

- Salt and pepper to taste

- 1/2 cup shredded mozzarella cheese

Directions:

1. Preheat the oven to 375°F (190°C).

2. In a skillet over medium heat, cook ground turkey and onion until the turkey is browned and the onion is soft.

3. Stir in cooked quinoa, spinach, tomato sauce, garlic powder, smoked paprika, salt, and pepper. Cook until the spinach is wilted.

4. Fill each bell pepper with the turkey and quinoa mixture. Place in a baking dish.

5. Cover with foil and bake for 25 minutes. Uncover, top each pepper with mozzarella cheese, and bake for an additional 5 minutes, or until the cheese is melted and bubbly.

6. Serve hot.

Nutrition Facts (per serving)

- Calories: 320
- Fat: 12g
- Carbohydrates: 22g
- Protein: 30g

Garlic Butter Chicken Thighs

Prep Time: 10 mins

Cook Time: 25 mins

Total Time: 35 mins

Servings: 4

Yield: 4 servings

Ingredients: 8 chicken thighs, bone-in and skin-on

- 4 tablespoons butter

- 3 garlic cloves, minced

- 1 teaspoon dried rosemary

- 1 teaspoon dried thyme

- Salt and pepper to taste

Directions:

1. Preheat the oven to 425°F (220°C).

2. In a skillet over medium heat, melt butter. Add garlic, rosemary, and thyme, cooking for 1-2 minutes until fragrant.

3. Season chicken thighs with salt and pepper. Add to the skillet, skin-side down, and cook until the skin is golden brown, about 5 minutes. Flip and cook for an additional 5 minutes.

4. Transfer the skillet to the oven and bake for 15-20 minutes, or until the chicken is cooked through and reaches an internal temperature of 165°F (74°C).

5. Serve hot, spooning the garlic butter sauce over the chicken.

Nutrition Facts (per serving)

- Calories: 450

- Fat: 35g

- Carbohydrates: 1g

- Protein: 35g

Zucchini Noodles with Pesto

Prep Time: 15 mins

Cook Time: 5 mins

Total Time: 20 mins

Servings: 4

Yield: 4 servings
Ingredients:

- 4 large zucchinis, spiralized

- 1 cup basil pesto, homemade or store-bought

- 1/2 cup cherry tomatoes, halved

- 1/4 cup pine nuts, toasted

- Salt and pepper to taste

- Grated Parmesan cheese, for serving

Directions:

1. In a large skillet over medium heat, cook spiralized zucchini noodles for 2-3 minutes, just until tender.

2. Remove from heat and stir in basil pesto until the noodles are well coated.

3. Add cherry tomatoes and toasted pine nuts. Season with salt and pepper.

4. Serve immediately, garnished with grated Parmesan cheese.

Nutrition Facts (per serving)

- Calories: 280

- Fat: 22g

- Carbohydrates: 10g

- Protein: 6g

Turkey Meatball Soup

Prep Time: 20 mins
Cook Time: 30 mins
Total Time: 50 mins
Servings: 6

Yield: 6 servings

Ingredients:

- 1 pound ground turkey
- 1/4 cup breadcrumbs
- 1 egg
- 2 tablespoons Parmesan cheese, grated
- 1 teaspoon garlic powder
- 1 teaspoon onion powder
- Salt and pepper to taste
- 1 tablespoon olive oil
- 6 cups chicken broth, low sodium
- 2 carrots, diced
- 2 celery stalks, diced
- 1 onion, diced
- 1 cup spinach, chopped

Directions:

1. In a bowl, mix together ground turkey, breadcrumbs, egg, Parmesan cheese, garlic powder, onion powder, salt, and pepper. Form into small meatballs.

2. Heat olive oil in a large pot over medium heat. Add meatballs and cook until browned on all sides. Remove meatballs from the pot.

3. In the same pot, add carrots, celery, and onion. Cook until vegetables are softened, about 5 minutes.

4. Pour in chicken broth and bring to a boil. Add meatballs back to the pot. Reduce heat and simmer for 20 minutes.

5. Stir in spinach and cook until wilted, about 2 minutes.

6. Serve hot.

Nutrition Facts (per serving)

- Calories: 220

- Fat: 10g

- Carbohydrates: 10g

- Protein: 25g

Grilled Lemon Herb Pork Chops

Prep Time: 15 mins (plus marinating time)

Cook Time: 12 mins

Total Time: 27 mins

Servings: 4

Yield: 4 servings

Ingredients:

- 4 pork chops, bone-in

- 2 lemons, juiced

- 2 tablespoons olive oil

- 2 garlic cloves, minced

- 1 teaspoon dried oregano

- 1 teaspoon dried basil

- Salt and pepper to taste

Directions:

1. In a bowl, whisk together lemon juice, olive oil, garlic, oregano, basil, salt, and pepper.

2. Place pork chops in a large resealable bag. Pour the marinade over the chops, seal the bag, and ensure each chop is well

coated. Marinate in the refrigerator for at least 1 hour, or overnight for best flavor.

3. Preheat grill to medium-high heat. Remove pork chops from marinade, discarding any excess marinade.

4. Grill pork chops for 5-6 minutes on each side, or until they reach an internal temperature of 145°F (63°C).

5. Let rest for 5 minutes before serving.

Nutrition Facts (per serving)

- Calories: 290

- Fat: 16g

- Carbohydrates: 3g

- Protein: 30g

Cauliflower Steak with Herb Sauce

Prep Time: 10 mins, Cook Time: 20 mins, Total Time: 30 mins

Servings: 4, Yield: 4 servings

Ingredients:

- 2 large heads cauliflower

- 3 tablespoons olive oil

- Salt and pepper to taste

For the Herb Sauce:

- 1/2 cup fresh parsley, chopped

- 1/4 cup fresh cilantro, chopped

- 2 tablespoons olive oil

- 1 tablespoon lemon juice

- 1 garlic clove, minced

- Salt and pepper to taste

Directions:

1. Preheat the oven to 400°F (200°C). Slice cauliflower heads into 1-inch thick steaks, yielding about 2 steaks per head.

2. Brush both sides of each cauliflower steak with olive oil and season with salt and pepper. Place on a baking sheet.

3. Roast in the preheated oven for 20 minutes, flipping halfway through, until tender and golden.

4. While the cauliflower roasts, prepare the herb sauce by mixing parsley, cilantro, olive oil, lemon juice, garlic, salt, and pepper in a bowl.

5. Serve cauliflower steaks drizzled with the herb sauce.

Nutrition Facts (per serving)

- Calories: 210
- Fat: 14g
- Carbohydrates: 18g
- Protein: 6g

Baked Tilapia with Dill Sauce

Prep Time: 5 mins

Cook Time: 15 mins

Total Time: 20 mins

Servings: 4

Yield: 4 servings

Ingredients: 4 tilapia fillets

- 2 tablespoons olive oil

- Salt and pepper to taste

For the Dill Sauce:

- 1/4 cup Greek yogurt

- 1 tablespoon fresh dill, chopped

- 1 teaspoon lemon juice

- 1 garlic clove, minced

- Salt and pepper to taste

Directions:

1. Preheat the oven to 375°F (190°C). Place tilapia fillets on a baking sheet. Brush each fillet with olive oil and season with salt and pepper.

2. Bake in the preheated oven for 12-15 minutes, or until fish flakes easily with a fork.

3. While the fish is baking, mix together Greek yogurt, dill, lemon juice, garlic, salt, and pepper in a bowl to create the dill sauce.

4. Serve the baked tilapia topped with dill sauce.

Nutrition Facts (per serving)

- Calories: 180

- Fat: 9g

- Carbohydrates: 1g

- Protein: 23g

Roasted Vegetable Quiche

Prep Time: 20 mins

Cook Time: 35 mins

Total Time: 55 mins

Servings: 6

Yield: 1 quiche

Ingredients:

- 1 pie crust, pre-made or homemade
- 2 cups mixed vegetables (e.g., bell peppers, zucchini, and onions), diced
- 1 tablespoon olive oil
- Salt and pepper to taste
- 4 large eggs
- 1 cup milk
- 1/2 cup shredded cheddar cheese
- 1 teaspoon dried thyme

Directions:

1. Preheat the oven to 375°F (190°C). Toss diced vegetables with olive oil, salt, and pepper. Spread on a baking sheet and roast for 15 minutes, until tender.

2. Whisk together eggs, milk, cheese, and thyme in a bowl. Season with salt and pepper.

3. Place the pre-baked pie crust on a baking sheet. Spread roasted vegetables evenly over the crust. Pour the egg mixture over the vegetables.

4. Bake in the preheated oven for 35-40 minutes, or until the quiche is set and the crust is golden brown.

5. Let cool for 10 minutes before slicing and serving.

Nutrition Facts (per serving)

- Calories: 280
- Fat: 18g

- Carbohydrates: 18g

- Protein: 12g

Lemon Garlic Roasted Chicken Breasts

Prep Time: 10 mins

Cook Time: 30 mins

Total Time: 40 mins

Servings: 4

Yield: 4 servings

Ingredients:

- 4 boneless, skinless chicken breasts

- 2 tablespoons olive oil

- 2 lemons, 1 juiced and 1 sliced

- 4 garlic cloves, minced

- 1 teaspoon dried rosemary

- Salt and pepper to taste

Directions:

1. Preheat the oven to 375°F (190°C).

2. In a small bowl, mix together olive oil, lemon juice, minced garlic, rosemary, salt, and pepper.

3. Place chicken breasts in a baking dish. Pour the lemon garlic mixture over the chicken, ensuring each piece is well coated. Arrange lemon slices around and on top of the chicken.

4. Bake in the preheated oven for 30 minutes, or until the chicken is cooked through and reaches an internal temperature of 165°F (74°C).

5. Serve hot, garnished with additional fresh rosemary if desired.

Nutrition Facts (per serving)

- Calories: 220
- Fat: 10g
- Carbohydrates: 3g
- Protein: 30g

Chickpea and Spinach Curry

Prep Time: 10 mins

Cook Time: 20 mins

Total Time: 30 mins

Servings: 4

Yield: 4 servings

Ingredients:

- 1 tablespoon olive oil
- 1 onion, diced
- 2 garlic cloves, minced
- 1 tablespoon curry powder
- 1 can (15 oz) chickpeas, drained and rinsed
- 1 can (14.5 oz) diced tomatoes, with juice
- 2 cups baby spinach leaves
- 1 cup coconut milk
- Salt and pepper to taste
- Cooked rice, for serving

Directions:

1. Heat olive oil in a large skillet over medium heat. Add onion and garlic, and sauté until softened, about 5 minutes.

2. Stir in curry powder and cook for 1 minute until fragrant.

3. Add chickpeas and diced tomatoes with their juice. Bring to a simmer and cook for 10 minutes.

4. Stir in baby spinach and coconut milk. Continue to cook until the spinach has wilted and the curry is heated through, about 5 minutes. Season with salt and pepper to taste.

5. Serve hot over cooked rice.

Nutrition Facts (per serving)

- Calories: 260
- Fat: 14g
- Carbohydrates: 28g
- Protein: 8g

SNACK

Cucumber Sandwiches

Prep Time: 10 mins

Cook Time: 0 mins

Total Time: 10 mins

Servings: 4

Yield: 8 sandwiches

Ingredients:

- 1 large cucumber, sliced thinly
- 4 ounces cream cheese, softened
- 2 tablespoons fresh dill, chopped
- 1/4 teaspoon garlic powder
- Salt and pepper to taste
- 8 slices of whole grain bread, crusts removed

Directions:

1. In a small bowl, mix together the cream cheese, dill, garlic powder, salt, and pepper until well combined.
2. Spread the cream cheese mixture on 4 slices of bread.
3. Arrange cucumber slices over the cream cheese.
4. Top with the remaining slices of bread, cut each sandwich into two triangles, and serve.

Nutrition Facts (per serving)

- Calories: 150
- Fat: 8g

- Carbohydrates: 15g

- Protein: 4g

Apple Peanut Butter Slices

Prep Time: 5 mins

Cook Time: 0 mins

Total Time: 5 mins

Servings: 2

Yield: 1 apple

Ingredients:

- 1 medium apple, cored and sliced

- 2 tablespoons peanut butter

Directions:

1. Spread peanut butter evenly over apple slices.

2. Serve immediately or chill in the refrigerator before serving.

Nutrition Facts (per serving)

- Calories: 180

- Fat: 8g

- Carbohydrates: 24g

- Protein: 4g

Carrot and Hummus Dip

Prep Time: 5 mins, Cook Time: 0 mins

Total Time: 5 mins

Servings: 4,

Yield: 2 cups

Ingredients: 2 cups baby carrots and 1/2 cup hummus

Directions: Serve baby carrots with hummus for dipping.

Nutrition Facts (per serving)

- Calories: 105

- Fat: 5g

- Carbohydrates: 12g

- Protein: 3g

Greek Yogurt with Berries

Prep Time: 5 mins

Cook Time: 0 mins

Total Time: 5 mins

Servings: 1

Yield: 1 serving

Ingredients: 1 cup plain Greek yogurt

- 1/2 cup mixed berries (strawberries, blueberries, raspberries)

Directions:

1. Top Greek yogurt with mixed berries.

2. Serve immediately.

Nutrition Facts (per serving)

- Calories: 150

- Fat: 1g

- Carbohydrates: 18g

- Protein: 20g

Cheese and Crackers

Prep Time: 5 mins

Cook Time: 0 mins

Total Time: 5 mins

Servings: 2

Yield: 4 crackers

Ingredients:

- 4 whole grain crackers
- 4 slices of cheddar cheese

Directions:

1. Place a slice of cheese on each cracker.
2. Serve immediately or chill in the refrigerator before serving.

Nutrition Facts (per serving)

- Calories: 200
- Fat: 12g
- Carbohydrates: 10g
- Protein: 10g

Turkey Roll-Ups

Prep Time: 10 mins

Cook Time: 0 mins

Total Time: 10 mins

Servings: 4

Yield: 8 roll-ups

Ingredients:

- 8 slices of turkey breast

- 4 sticks of low-fat string cheese

- 1/4 cup spinach leaves

Directions:

1. Lay out turkey slices. Place a stick of string cheese and a few spinach leaves on each slice.

2. Roll up tightly and serve.

Nutrition Facts (per serving)

- Calories: 120

- Fat: 4g

- Carbohydrates: 1g

- Protein: 20g

Almond Butter Celery Sticks

Prep Time: 5 mins

Cook Time: 0 mins

Total Time: 5 mins

Servings: 2

Yield: 4 sticks

Ingredients:

- 4 celery sticks, trimmed

- 2 tablespoons almond butter

Directions:

1. Fill each celery stick with almond butter.

2. Serve immediately or chill before serving.

Nutrition Facts (per serving)

- Calories: 98
- Fat: 8g
- Carbohydrates: 4g
- Protein: 3g

Cottage Cheese and Pineapple

Prep Time: 5 mins

Cook Time: 0 mins

Total Time: 5 mins

Servings: 1

Yield: 1 serving

Ingredients:

- 1/2 cup low-fat cottage cheese
- 1/2 cup pineapple chunks

Directions:

1. Mix cottage cheese with pineapple chunks.
2. Serve chilled.

Nutrition Facts (per serving)

- Calories: 120
- Fat: 1g
- Carbohydrates: 15g
- Protein: 12g

Baked Kale Chips

Prep Time: 10 mins

Cook Time: 15 mins

Total Time: 25 mins

Servings: 2

Yield: 2 cups

Ingredients:

- 2 cups kale leaves, washed and dried

- 1 tablespoon olive oil

- Salt to taste

Directions:

1. Preheat the oven to 350°F (175°C).

2. Toss kale leaves with olive oil and salt. Spread on a baking sheet in a single layer.

3. Bake for 15 minutes, or until crisp.

4. Serve immediately.

Nutrition Facts (per serving)

- Calories: 80

- Fat: 7g

- Carbohydrates: 5g

- Protein: 2g

DESSERT

Berry Almond Crisp

Prep Time: 15 mins
Cook Time: 30 mins
Total Time: 45 mins
Servings: 6
Yield: 1 crisp

Ingredients:

- 2 cups mixed berries (strawberries, blueberries, raspberries)
- 1 tablespoon granulated sugar
- 1 teaspoon vanilla extract
- 3/4 cup rolled oats
- 1/4 cup almond flour
- 1/4 cup sliced almonds
- 1/4 cup unsalted butter, melted
- 2 tablespoons honey

Directions:

1. Preheat the oven to 375°F (190°C) and grease a baking dish.

2. In a bowl, mix together berries, sugar, and vanilla extract. Spread the berry mixture in the prepared baking dish.

3. In another bowl, combine rolled oats, almond flour, sliced almonds, melted butter, and honey. Mix until crumbly.

4. Sprinkle the oat mixture over the berries.

5. Bake in the preheated oven for 30 minutes or until the topping is golden and the berries are bubbly.

6. Serve warm or at room temperature.

Nutrition Facts (per serving)

- Calories: 220

- Fat: 12g

- Carbohydrates: 26g

- Protein: 4g

Vanilla Chia Pudding

Prep Time: *5 mins, Cook Time: 0 mins (Refrigerate for 4 hours)*
Total Time*: 4 hours 5 mins*
Serving*s: 4*
Yield*: 4 servings*
Ingredients: 2 cups almond milk

- 1/2 cup chia seeds

- 2 tablespoons maple syrup

- 1 teaspoon vanilla extract

Directions:

1. In a bowl, whisk together almond milk, chia seeds, maple syrup, and vanilla extract until well combined.

2. Divide the mixture among four serving glasses or bowls.

3. Refrigerate for at least 4 hours, or until the pudding has thickened.

4. Serve chilled, topped with fresh berries if desired.

Nutrition Facts (per serving)

- Calories: 180

- Fat: 9g

- Carbohydrates: 20g

- Protein: 5g

Peach Sorbet

Prep Time: *10 mins*
Cook Time: *0 mins (Freeze for 4 hours)*
Total Time: *4 hours 10 mins*
Servings: *4*
Yield: *4 servings*
Ingredients: 4 cups frozen peaches

- 1/4 cup honey

- 2 tablespoons lemon juice

Directions:

1. In a blender, combine frozen peaches, honey, and lemon juice. Blend until smooth.

2. Transfer the mixture to a freezer-safe container.

3. Freeze for at least 4 hours, or until firm.

4. Serve scoops of sorbet garnished with fresh mint leaves.

Nutrition Facts (per serving)

- Calories: 160

- Fat: 0g

- Carbohydrates: 40g

- Protein: 2g

Coconut Macaroons

Prep Time: *15 mins*
Cook Time: *15 mins*
Total Time: *30 mins*

Servings: 6
Yield: 12 macaroons
Ingredients:

- 2 cups shredded unsweetened coconut

- 3 large egg whites

- 1/4 cup granulated sugar

- 1 teaspoon vanilla extract

- Pinch of salt

Directions:

1. Preheat the oven to 325°F (165°C) and line a baking sheet with parchment paper.

2. In a bowl, mix together coconut, egg whites, sugar, vanilla extract, and a pinch of salt.

3. Drop tablespoonfuls of the mixture onto the prepared baking sheet, forming small mounds.

4. Bake in the preheated oven for 15 minutes or until golden.

5. Let cool on the baking sheet before serving.

Nutrition Facts (per serving)

- Calories: 200

- Fat: 15g

- Carbohydrates: 15g

- Protein: 3g

Apple Cinnamon Baked Oatmeal Cups

*Prep Time: 15 mins, **Cook Time:** 25 mins*
Total Time: 40 mins
Servings: 6

Yield: *12 oatmeal cups*

Ingredients:

- 3 cups rolled oats
- 1 teaspoon baking powder
- 2 teaspoons cinnamon
- 1/4 teaspoon salt
- 1 cup unsweetened applesauce
- 1/2 cup milk
- 1/4 cup maple syrup
- 1 large egg
- 1 teaspoon vanilla extract
- 1 cup diced apples

Directions:

1. Preheat the oven to 375°F (190°C) and grease a muffin tin.
2. In a large bowl, mix together oats, baking powder, cinnamon, and salt.
3. In another bowl, whisk together applesauce, milk, maple syrup, egg, and vanilla extract.
4. Combine the wet ingredients with the dry ingredients, then fold in the diced apples.
5. Divide the mixture evenly among the muffin cups.
6. Bake in the preheated oven for 25 minutes or until set and golden on top.
7. Let cool before serving.

Nutrition Facts (per serving)

- Calories: 220

- Fat: 3g

- Carbohydrates: 42g

- Protein: 6g

Strawberry Yogurt Popsicles

Prep Time: *10 mins*
Cook Time: *0 mins (Freeze for 4 hours)*
Total Time: *4 hours 10 mins*
Servings: *6*
Yield: *6 popsicles*

Ingredients:

- 2 cups fresh strawberries, hulled

- 1 cup plain Greek yogurt

- 2 tablespoons honey

Directions:

1. In a blender, puree strawberries, Greek yogurt, and honey until smooth.

2. Pour the mixture into popsicle molds, insert sticks, and freeze for at least 4 hours, or until solid.

3. To serve, run warm water over the outside of the molds for a few seconds to easily release the popsicles.

Nutrition Facts (per serving)

- Calories: 80

- Fat: 0.5g

- Carbohydrates: 14g

- Protein: 5g

Almond Flour Shortbread Cookies

Prep Time: *15 mins*
Cook Time: *12 mins*
Total Time: *27 mins*
Servings: *6*
Yield: *12 cookies*

Ingredients:

- 2 cups almond flour

- 1/3 cup granulated sugar

- 1/4 teaspoon salt

- 1/2 cup unsalted butter, softened

- 1 teaspoon vanilla extract

Directions:

1. Preheat the oven to 350°F (175°C) and line a baking sheet with parchment paper.

2. In a bowl, mix together almond flour, sugar, and salt. Add butter and vanilla extract, mixing until a dough forms.

3. Roll the dough into 1-inch balls and place on the prepared baking sheet. Flatten slightly with the back of a fork.

4. Bake in the preheated oven for 12 minutes or until the edges are golden brown.

5. Let cool on the baking sheet before transferring to a wire rack to cool completely.

Nutrition Facts (per serving)

- Calories: 280

- Fat: 23g

- Carbohydrates: 14g

- Protein: 6g

Baked Pear with Cinnamon and Honey

Prep Time: 5 mins
Cook Time: 25 mins
Total Time: 30 mins
Servings: 4
Yield: 4 servings

Ingredients:

- 2 large pears, halved and cored
- 2 tablespoons honey
- 1/2 teaspoon cinnamon
- 1/4 cup chopped walnuts

Directions:

1. Preheat the oven to 350°F (175°C). Place pear halves cut-side up on a baking dish.
2. Drizzle honey over each pear half and sprinkle with cinnamon. Top with chopped walnuts.
3. Bake in the preheated oven for 25 minutes, or until pears are tender.
4. Serve warm, with a dollop of Greek yogurt if desired.

Nutrition Facts (per serving)

- Calories: 150
- Fat: 5g
- Carbohydrates: 27g
- Protein: 2g

Chocolate Avocado Mousse

Prep Time: *10 mins*
Cook Time: *0 mins*
Total Time: *10 mins*
Servings: *4*
Yield: *4 servings*
Ingredients:

- 2 ripe avocados, peeled and pitted
- 1/4 cup cocoa powder
- 1/4 cup honey
- 1/2 teaspoon vanilla extract
- A pinch of salt

Directions:

1. In a blender or food processor, combine avocados, cocoa powder, honey, vanilla extract, and a pinch of salt. Blend until smooth and creamy.
2. Divide the mousse among serving dishes and refrigerate for at least 1 hour before serving.
3. Garnish with fresh berries or a sprinkle of cocoa powder before serving.

Nutrition Facts (per serving)

- Calories: 230
- Fat: 15g
- Carbohydrates: 27g
- Protein: 3g

Raspberry Lemon Bars

Prep Time: 15 mins
Cook Time: 35 mins
Total Time: 50 mins
Servings: 8
Yield: 8 bars

Ingredients:

For the crust:

- 1 cup almond flour
- 1/4 cup coconut flour
- 1/4 cup unsalted butter, melted
- 2 tablespoons honey

For the filling:

- 3 large eggs
- 1/2 cup honey
- 1/2 cup lemon juice
- 2 teaspoons lemon zest
- 1 cup fresh raspberries

Directions:

1. Preheat the oven to 350°F (175°C) and line an 8x8-inch baking pan with parchment paper.

2. Mix almond flour, coconut flour, melted butter, and honey in a bowl. Press the mixture into the bottom of the prepared pan to form a crust.

3. Bake the crust for 10 minutes, then remove from the oven.

4. In a bowl, whisk together eggs, honey, lemon juice, and lemon zest. Gently fold in raspberries. Pour the filling over the baked crust.

5. Return to the oven and bake for an additional 25 minutes, or until the filling is set.

6. Let cool completely before cutting into bars. Serve chilled.

Nutrition Facts (per serving)

- Calories: 280

- Fat: 15g

- Carbohydrates: 34g

- Protein: 6g

MEAL PLAN

Day 1

Breakfast: Apple Cinnamon Oatmeal

Lunch: Turkey and Avocado Salad

Dinner: Lemon Herb Baked Cod

Day 2

Breakfast: Greek Yogurt with Berries

Lunch: Quinoa Vegetable Soup

Dinner: Grilled Chicken and Vegetable Kabobs

Day 3

Breakfast: Berry Smoothie Bowl

Lunch: Beef and Broccoli Stir-Fry

Dinner: Spaghetti Squash with Tomato Basil Sauce

Day 4

Breakfast: Vanilla Chia Pudding

Lunch: Chicken Caesar Salad Wrap

Dinner: Baked Tilapia with Dill Sauce

Day 5

Breakfast: Peanut Butter and Banana Sandwich

Lunch: Mediterranean Quinoa Salad

Dinner: Zucchini Noodles with Pesto

Day 6

Breakfast: Cottage Cheese with Pineapple

Lunch: Grilled Lemon Herb Pork Chops

Dinner: Roasted Vegetable Quiche

Day 7

Breakfast: Veggie Egg Muffins

Lunch: Stuffed Bell Peppers

Dinner: Garlic Butter Chicken Thighs

Day 8

Breakfast: Almond Butter Celery Sticks

Lunch: Tuna Salad Stuffed Avocado

Dinner: Chicken and Rice Soup

Day 9

Breakfast: Cucumber Sandwiches

Lunch: Turkey Roll-Ups

Dinner: Spinach and Cheese Stuffed Chicken

Day 10

Breakfast: Cheese and Crackers

Lunch: Shrimp and Asparagus Salad

Dinner: Lemon Garlic Roasted Chicken Breasts

Day 11

Breakfast: Baked Kale Chips

Lunch: Spinach and Feta Omelette

Dinner: Chickpea and Spinach Curry

Day 12

Breakfast: Zucchini Muffins

Lunch: Avocado Toast with Egg

Dinner: Coconut Macaroons

Day 13

Breakfast: Strawberry Yogurt Popsicles

Lunch: Greek Yogurt Parfait

Dinner: Almond Flour Shortbread Cookies

Day 14

Breakfast: Baked Pear with Cinnamon and Honey

Lunch: Raspberry Lemon Bars

Dinner: Chocolate Avocado Mousse

Day 15

Breakfast: Apple Peanut Butter Slices

Lunch: Carrot and Hummus Dip

Dinner: Peach Sorbet

Day 16

Breakfast: Greek Yogurt with Berries

Lunch: Chicken Caesar Salad Wrap

Dinner: Zucchini Noodles with Pesto

Day 17

Breakfast: Veggie Egg Muffins

Lunch: Quinoa Vegetable Soup

Dinner: Lemon Herb Baked Cod

Day 18

Breakfast: Berry Smoothie Bowl

Lunch: Turkey and Avocado Salad

Dinner: Garlic Butter Chicken Thighs

Day 19

Breakfast: Vanilla Chia Pudding

Lunch: Mediterranean Quinoa Salad

Dinner: Grilled Lemon Herb Pork Chops

Day 20

Breakfast: Cottage Cheese with Pineapple

Lunch: Beef and Broccoli Stir-Fry

Dinner: Chicken and Rice Soup

Day 21

Breakfast: Peanut Butter and Banana Sandwich

Lunch: Stuffed Bell Peppers

Dinner: Spinach and Cheese Stuffed Chicken

Day 22

Breakfast: Apple Cinnamon Oatmeal

Lunch: Shrimp and Asparagus Salad

Dinner: Spaghetti Squash with Tomato Basil Sauce

Day 23

Breakfast: Cucumber Sandwiches

Lunch: Tuna Salad Stuffed Avocado

Dinner: Baked Tilapia with Dill Sauce

Day 24

Breakfast: Cheese and Crackers

Lunch: Turkey Roll-Ups

Dinner: Roasted Vegetable Quiche

Day 25

Breakfast: Almond Butter Celery Sticks

Lunch: Avocado Toast with Egg

Dinner: Lemon Garlic Roasted Chicken Breasts

Day 26

Breakfast: Strawberry Yogurt Popsicles

Lunch: Greek Yogurt Parfait

Dinner: Chickpea and Spinach Curry

Day 27

Breakfast: Baked Kale Chips

Lunch: Raspberry Lemon Bars

Dinner: Chocolate Avocado Mousse

Day 28

Breakfast: Zucchini Muffins

Lunch: Carrot and Hummus Dip

Dinner: Peach Sorbet

MANAGING POTASSIUM LEVELS AND HEALTH

Managing Potassium Levels and Health

Potassium, a vital mineral, plays a crucial role in maintaining several bodily functions, including the regulation of heart rhythm, muscle contraction, and nerve signals. Despite its importance, maintaining the right balance of potassium is a delicate dance for many, especially those with certain health conditions. This chapter delves into the intricacies of monitoring potassium levels, recognizing the symptoms of hyperkalemia, and implementing strategies to prevent high potassium episodes.

Monitoring Potassium Levels

Understanding the Importance of Potassium Balance

Potassium balance is essential for health, influencing heart function, muscle work, and nerve cell communication. The body meticulously regulates potassium levels, but certain conditions and medications can disrupt this balance, necessitating regular monitoring.

Methods for Monitoring Potassium Levels

The primary method for assessing potassium levels is through blood tests, which provide a direct measure of the amount of potassium in the bloodstream. For individuals at risk of hyperkalemia, regular blood tests are crucial. These tests are typically part of routine health checks, especially for those with kidney disease, heart conditions, or on specific medications that affect potassium levels.

Interpreting Potassium Levels

Normal blood potassium levels are generally between 3.6 and 5.2 millimoles per liter (mmol/L). Levels above 5.5 mmol/L may indicate hyperkalemia, necessitating further investigation and management. It's important for patients and healthcare providers to understand these values, as they guide dietary recommendations and medication adjustments.

Understanding the Symptoms of High Potassium (Hyperkalemia)

Recognizing the Signs and Symptoms

Hyperkalemia often remains asymptomatic until potassium levels become significantly elevated. Symptoms can include muscle weakness, fatigue, palpitations, and, in severe cases, life-threatening heart rhythm problems. Early recognition of these symptoms is crucial for prompt management and prevention of complications.

The Health Implications of Hyperkalemia

High potassium levels can have serious health implications, particularly for the cardiovascular system. In extreme cases, hyperkalemia can lead to cardiac arrest. The risk is higher in individuals with underlying heart conditions or those taking medications that increase potassium levels.

When to Seek Medical Attention

Anyone experiencing symptoms suggestive of hyperkalemia, especially those with risk factors for elevated potassium levels, should seek immediate medical attention. Early intervention can prevent serious complications and help manage the condition effectively.

Strategies for Preventing High Potassium Episodes

Dietary Management

Diet plays a pivotal role in managing potassium levels. A dietitian can provide tailored advice, identifying foods high in potassium that should be limited or avoided. This includes certain fruits, vegetables, dairy products, and whole grains. Instead, a focus on low-potassium foods can help maintain balance without compromising nutritional intake.

Medication Management

Certain medications can increase potassium levels, including some blood pressure medications, like ACE inhibitors and potassium-sparing diuretics. Regular review of medication by a healthcare provider is essential to identify any potential impacts on potassium levels and adjust treatment as necessary.

Lifestyle Modifications

In addition to dietary changes, lifestyle modifications can contribute to maintaining optimal potassium levels. This includes staying hydrated, managing chronic conditions effectively, and avoiding excessive use of potassium supplements.

Regular Monitoring and Health Checks

For those at risk of hyperkalemia, regular health checks and blood tests are crucial. These checks help monitor potassium levels over time, allowing for early detection of changes and adjustments in management strategies.

SPECIAL CONSIDERATIONS FOR WOMEN

Women's bodies undergo various physiological changes throughout their lives, from menstrual cycles to pregnancy and menopause. These changes can significantly impact nutritional needs, including potassium levels, which play a crucial role in maintaining overall health. This chapter delves into how hormonal changes affect potassium levels, considerations for a low potassium diet during pregnancy, and the relationship between menopause and potassium regulation.

How Hormonal Changes Affect Potassium Levels

The Impact of the Menstrual Cycle

The menstrual cycle can influence potassium levels in the body. During the luteal phase of the menstrual cycle, some women may experience changes in fluid and electrolyte balance, leading to variations in potassium levels. These fluctuations can contribute to symptoms such as bloating and mood swings. A balanced diet, rich in a variety of nutrients, can help mitigate these effects and maintain stable potassium levels throughout the cycle.

Hormonal Contraceptives and Potassium

Hormonal contraceptives, such as the pill, patch, or ring, can also impact potassium levels. Some forms of hormonal birth control can lead to an increase in potassium, necessitating careful monitoring in women with existing health conditions that affect potassium regulation, such as kidney disease. Women using these contraceptives should discuss their potassium levels with their healthcare provider to ensure they remain within a healthy range.

Managing Potassium Levels Through Diet

A diet that carefully considers potassium intake can help manage these hormonal effects. Incorporating a variety of fruits, vegetables, lean proteins, and whole grains, while monitoring high-potassium foods, can support women's health throughout the menstrual cycle and when using hormonal contraceptives. Regular blood tests may be recommended for those at risk of potassium imbalances to tailor dietary recommendations further.

Pregnancy and Low Potassium Diet Considerations

The Importance of Potassium During Pregnancy

Potassium plays a vital role in supporting a healthy pregnancy, contributing to muscle function, nerve signals, and fluid balance. However, maintaining the right balance is key. Both high and low potassium levels can have implications for maternal and fetal health, making monitoring and management essential.

Dietary Recommendations for Pregnant Women

Pregnant women should aim for a balanced diet that meets their increased nutritional needs without excessively elevating potassium levels. Foods rich in potassium, such as bananas, oranges, and potatoes, should be consumed in moderation. At the same time, adequate intake of other essential nutrients must be ensured to support fetal development and maternal health.

Monitoring and Adjustments

Regular prenatal check-ups will include blood tests to monitor potassium levels, among other vital nutrients. Any dietary adjustments should be made under the guidance of a healthcare provider or a registered dietitian to ensure the health and safety of both the mother and the developing fetus.

Menopause and Potassium Regulation

Changes in Potassium Needs After Menopause

Menopause marks the end of a woman's reproductive years and brings about significant hormonal changes that can affect overall health, including potassium regulation. Postmenopausal women may experience changes in blood pressure and bone density, in which potassium plays a role. Ensuring adequate potassium intake can support cardiovascular health and may help prevent osteoporosis.

Dietary Strategies for Postmenopausal Women

A diet rich in fruits, vegetables, lean proteins, and whole grains can help manage potassium levels and support overall health during menopause. Foods that are high in antioxidants and low in sodium can also benefit cardiovascular health. Calcium and vitamin D are particularly important for bone health, while potassium can aid in their absorption and utilization.

Lifestyle and Nutritional Considerations

In addition to dietary management, regular physical activity, stress reduction techniques, and adequate hydration are important for managing health during menopause. Women should work with their healthcare providers to monitor their health, including potassium levels, and make any necessary adjustments to their diet and lifestyle to support their well-being during this transition.

EXERCISE AND LOW POTASSIUM DIET

For women on a low potassium diet, the interplay between diet, potassium levels, and exercise is nuanced. Potassium, a critical electrolyte, plays a pivotal role in muscle function, nerve signals, and fluid balance in the body. During exercise, potassium levels fluctuate as muscles contract and relax, and the body loses electrolytes through sweat. Thus, managing potassium intake and understanding its dynamics during physical activity is crucial for women on a restricted potassium regimen.

Exercise Guidelines for Women on a Low Potassium Diet

1. Consultation with Healthcare Providers

Before embarking on an exercise regimen, it's imperative for women on a low potassium diet to consult with healthcare professionals. This consultation should aim to assess overall health, understand the specific dietary restrictions, and determine any potential risks associated with exercise. A tailored exercise plan can then be developed, taking into consideration individual health status, fitness level, and potassium management needs.

2. Hydration and Electrolyte Balance

Hydration is paramount during exercise, more so for individuals managing potassium levels. Women should focus on staying well-hydrated before, during, and after physical activity. However, caution is advised regarding electrolyte-replacement beverages, as many contain high levels of potassium. Opting for low-potassium hydration options or simply water, and consulting a dietitian for personalized advice on electrolyte management during exercise, is recommended.

3. Gradual Intensity Increase

For those new to exercise or returning after a hiatus, gradually increasing the intensity and duration of workouts is key. Starting with low-impact activities such as walking, yoga, or swimming can help the body adjust without overwhelming the system. Incremental increases allow for monitoring of how the body, particularly muscle function and heart rate, responds to exercise under potassium dietary restrictions.

4. Regular Monitoring

Monitoring signs and symptoms of potassium imbalance is crucial, especially during the initial phases of an exercise regimen. Symptoms such as muscle weakness, cramping, or palpitations should not be ignored, as they may indicate electrolyte imbalances. Keeping a log of exercise activities, dietary intake, and any symptoms can be beneficial for healthcare providers to review and adjust guidelines as necessary.

5. Strength Training and Cardiovascular Health

Incorporating a mix of strength training and cardiovascular exercises can offer comprehensive health benefits, including improved muscle strength, bone density, and heart health. Strength training exercises, performed with caution and under professional guidance, can help build muscle without excessively taxing the system. Cardiovascular activities, tailored to individual fitness levels, support heart health and can be adjusted based on potassium management needs.

6. Rest and Recovery

Adequate rest and recovery are essential components of an exercise regimen, particularly for women managing potassium levels through diet. Rest days allow the body to recover, muscles to repair, and electrolyte levels to stabilize. Incorporating practices such as stretching, mindfulness, or light yoga on rest days can further support overall well-being.

7. Personalized Exercise Regimen

Tailor Exercise to Individual Health Status: It's crucial that exercise routines are personalized. Women should consider their current health status, including any existing conditions that might affect or be affected by exercise, such as kidney function or cardiovascular health. Working with a fitness professional who understands the implications of a low potassium diet can help in designing an exercise program that meets individual needs and goals.

8. Focus on Flexibility and Balance

Incorporate Flexibility and Balance Training: Exercises that enhance flexibility and balance are particularly beneficial, as they are less likely to cause significant shifts in potassium levels compared to high-intensity workouts. Activities like Pilates, tai chi, and certain forms of yoga not only improve flexibility and balance but also contribute to stress reduction and mental well-being, making them excellent additions to any exercise regimen.

9. Monitor Dietary Intake Around Exercise

Adjust Dietary Intake Based on Exercise Demands: The relationship between diet and exercise is dynamic. Women on a low potassium diet should pay close attention to their meal composition before and after workouts. Consuming a balanced meal with adequate carbohydrates and protein post-exercise can support muscle recovery without compromising potassium restrictions. Consulting with a dietitian can provide insights into the best dietary practices surrounding exercise sessions.

10. Listen to Your Body

Prioritize Listening to Your Body: The importance of tuning into one's body cannot be overstated. Women should be vigilant about recognizing and responding to their body's signals during and after exercise. If an activity feels overly strenuous or if unusual symptoms arise, it's important to pause and reassess. Adapting exercise routines based on how one feels can prevent potential health issues and ensure a positive and nurturing exercise experience.

11. Regular Review and Adjustment

Engage in Regular Reviews of Exercise and Health Status: Health and fitness are not static; they evolve over time. Regularly reviewing and adjusting exercise routines in consultation with healthcare and fitness professionals ensures that the exercise regimen remains aligned with current health status, potassium management goals, and overall wellness objectives. This may include periodic reassessments of fitness levels, health check-ups to monitor potassium levels, and discussions about any new or changing symptoms.

Pre- and Post-Workout Nutrition Tips

Pre-Workout Nutrition

The primary aim of pre-workout nutrition is to prepare the body for the demands of physical activity. This involves consuming foods that provide a steady source of energy, enhance endurance, and maintain hydration. For individuals on a low potassium diet, it's crucial to select foods that are not only energizing but also align with their dietary restrictions.

Carbohydrates are the body's preferred energy source during exercise. Complex carbohydrates, found in whole grains and certain fruits and vegetables with lower potassium content, such as apples, berries, and carrots, provide a sustained energy release. Consuming a small, carbohydrate-rich snack or meal about 1 to 3 hours before exercise can help ensure that energy levels remain stable throughout the workout.

Protein intake before exercise supports muscle function and can help prevent muscle damage. Lean protein sources, such as chicken breast, turkey, or low-fat dairy products, are excellent choices. For those on a low potassium diet, it's important to choose protein sources that are not only low in potassium but also easily digestible to avoid gastrointestinal discomfort during exercise.

Hydration is another critical component of pre-workout nutrition. Adequate fluid intake is essential for maintaining blood volume, regulating body temperature, and ensuring muscle function. While water is the most straightforward hydration choice, individuals who are exercising for prolonged periods may benefit from a low-potassium electrolyte solution to help replace lost electrolytes without exceeding their potassium limits.

Post-Workout Nutrition

The focus of post-workout nutrition is on recovery and replenishment. After exercise, the body needs to repair muscle tissues, replenish glycogen stores, and rehydrate.

Protein is again crucial in the post-workout phase, aiding in the repair of exercise-induced damage to muscle fibers. Consuming protein after exercise provides the amino acids necessary for muscle repair and growth. Options like whey protein isolate or plant-based proteins can be good choices, depending on individual dietary restrictions and preferences.

Carbohydrates help replenish the glycogen stores that have been depleted during exercise. Choosing low-potassium carbohydrates such as white rice, bread, and certain fruits can help restore glycogen levels effectively without impacting potassium levels adversely.

Rehydration is vital after exercise to replace fluids lost through sweat. Water should be the primary focus, but depending on the intensity and duration of the workout, incorporating a low-potassium electrolyte solution can help restore electrolyte balance. Monitoring urine color can be a practical approach to assessing hydration status, aiming for a pale straw color as an indicator of proper hydration.

Timing is also an essential factor in post-workout nutrition. The body is most receptive to replenishment within 30 to 45 minutes after exercise, often referred to as the "anabolic window." Consuming a mix of protein and carbohydrates during this time can maximize recovery and muscle synthesis.

Hydration and Electrolyte Balance

Fundamental components of ideal health and performance are electrolyte balance and hydration, particularly for those who exercise often. This delicate balance is necessary for maintaining physiological activities, including muscle contraction, nerve transmission, and fluid management throughout the body. Particularly in the context of exercise and general wellness, having a thorough understanding of the dynamics of electrolyte management and hydration can empower people to make wise decisions regarding their nutrition and hydration strategies.

The Role of Hydration

Water is the most abundant substance in the human body, playing a pivotal role in various physiological processes. It serves as a medium for cellular reactions, aids in temperature regulation through sweating, transports nutrients and waste products, and acts as a lubricant and cushion for joints and tissues. Adequate hydration is essential for these processes to function optimally.

Dehydration, even in its mild form, can lead to a decline in physical performance, cognitive function, and overall well-being. Symptoms of dehydration include thirst, reduced urine output, dark-colored urine, fatigue, dizziness, and confusion. These signs indicate the body's need for fluids and should prompt immediate action to rehydrate.

Understanding Electrolytes

Electrolytes, including sodium, potassium, calcium, magnesium, chloride, phosphate, and bicarbonate, are minerals that carry an electric charge when dissolved in body fluids. These charged particles are critical for maintaining the electrical gradients across cell membranes, which are necessary for muscle contractions, heartbeat regulation, and neurological functions.

The balance of electrolytes in the body is tightly regulated, but it can be disrupted by factors such as excessive sweating, inadequate dietary intake, and certain medical conditions. Imbalances can lead to a range of issues, from muscle cramps and weakness to severe complications like arrhythmias and neurological disturbances.

Hydration Strategies

To maintain hydration, it is recommended to consume fluids regularly throughout the day, not just when thirst is perceived. The amount of fluid required depends on various factors, including age, gender, weight, climate, and activity level. As a general guideline, consuming at least 8-10 glasses (about 2 liters) of water daily is advised, with additional intake before, during, and after exercise.

For activities lasting less than an hour, water is typically sufficient to maintain hydration. However, for prolonged or intense exercise, especially in hot and humid conditions, sports drinks containing electrolytes and carbohydrates can be beneficial. These beverages help replenish electrolytes lost through sweat and provide energy to sustain performance.

Electrolyte Management

Maintaining electrolyte balance involves more than just managing sodium and potassium levels; it requires a holistic approach to nutrition. A diet rich in fruits, vegetables, whole grains, and lean proteins can provide the necessary minerals to support electrolyte balance. For individuals with specific dietary restrictions or those at risk of electrolyte imbalances, consulting with a healthcare provider or a dietitian can help tailor dietary plans to meet individual needs.

In cases of significant electrolyte imbalances, medical intervention may be necessary. Supplements or intravenous electrolyte solutions can be administered under medical supervision to quickly restore balance and prevent complications.

MENTAL AND EMOTIONAL WELL-BEING

Managing the complexity of dietary restrictions has a substantial influence on our mental and emotional health in addition to requiring us to make nutritional adjustments. Maintaining a balanced and healthy lifestyle requires knowing how to deal with these changes, getting assistance, and practicing stress reduction and mindfulness. This chapter explores these facets and provides information and techniques to assist people on their dietary journey.

Coping with Dietary Restrictions

Understanding the Emotional Impact

Dietary restrictions, whether for managing health conditions, allergies, or personal choices, can lead to feelings of isolation, frustration, and even grief. The sudden need to avoid certain foods that were once enjoyed can be challenging, impacting social interactions and personal satisfaction. Recognizing these feelings as valid and understandable is the first step in coping with dietary changes.

Strategies for Adaptation

Adapting to dietary restrictions involves more than just finding substitute ingredients; it's about redefining one's relationship with food. Here are strategies to facilitate this transition:

- **Education and Exploration:** Learning about your dietary needs can empower you to make informed choices. Exploring new recipes and foods can turn dietary restrictions into an opportunity for culinary creativity and discovery.

- **Setting Realistic Goals:** Start with small, achievable changes and gradually incorporate more as you become comfortable. Celebrate these milestones to motivate continued progress.

- **Focusing on Abundance:** Instead of focusing on what's missing, concentrate on the variety of foods you can enjoy. This shift in perspective can help alleviate feelings of deprivation.

Building Resilience

Resilience in the face of dietary restrictions comes from acknowledging the challenges and actively seeking solutions. Engaging in hobbies, connecting with nature, or practicing gratitude can enhance emotional resilience, providing a buffer against the stress of dietary management.

Seeking Support for Dietary Changes

The Role of Social Support

Social support is invaluable when navigating dietary changes. Sharing experiences, challenges, and successes with others who understand can significantly reduce feelings of isolation and stress. Support can come from various sources, including family, friends, support groups, or online communities.

Professional Guidance

Consulting with healthcare professionals such as dietitians, nutritionists, and therapists can provide tailored advice and emotional support. These experts can offer practical dietary strategies, coping mechanisms, and emotional support to navigate the complexities of dietary restrictions.

Creating a Supportive Environment

Educating those around you about your dietary needs can help create a supportive environment. Whether it's sharing safe recipes with family members or discussing restaurant options with friends, open communication is key to ensuring support from your social circle.

Mindfulness and Stress Management Techniques

The Power of Mindfulness

Mindfulness involves being present and fully engaged with the current moment, without judgment. This practice can be particularly beneficial for individuals dealing with dietary restrictions, as it encourages a non-judgmental acceptance of one's dietary journey.

Techniques for Practice

- **Mindful Eating:** Pay attention to the flavors, textures, and sensations of eating. This practice can enhance the enjoyment of food and promote a healthier relationship with eating.

- **Breathing Exercises:** Simple breathing techniques can help reduce stress and anxiety. Taking deep, controlled breaths can provide a sense of calm and relaxation.

- **Guided Imagery:** Visualizing peaceful scenes or positive outcomes can help manage stress and create a sense of well-being.

Incorporating Routine

Making mindfulness and stress management techniques a regular part of your routine can enhance their effectiveness. Whether it's starting the day with meditation, practicing breathing exercises during breaks, or engaging in mindful eating at meals, consistency is key.

CONCLUSION

Having taken a thorough tour from the first few pages of this book, we have now covered all of the fundamental areas of dietary control, with a particular emphasis on the nuances of being low in potassium. This story carefully led readers through the many facets of nutritional health, stressing the vital function potassium plays in our general well-being. It starts with an insightful introduction that lays the groundwork for the in-depth investigation to come.

The journey commenced with a foundational understanding of potassium's significance in "Understanding Potassium's Role in Women's Health," laying the groundwork for the discussions that followed. This initial exploration into the mineral's importance in bodily functions provided a crucial backdrop for the detailed guidance on managing potassium levels effectively, highlighting the delicate balance required for optimal health.

As we ventured into "Monitoring Potassium Levels," the narrative delved into practical strategies for keeping track of potassium intake, underscoring the importance of regular health checks and the implications of potassium imbalances. This section served as a cornerstone, equipping readers with the knowledge to navigate their dietary choices with confidence.

Progressing to "Exercise Guidelines for Women on a Low Potassium Diet," the book offered a nuanced look at how physical activity intersects with dietary management. This chapter emphasized the importance of tailoring exercise routines to complement a low potassium diet, ensuring that readers could maintain their physical health without compromising their dietary needs.

In "Hydration and Electrolyte Balance," the discussion expanded to the vital aspects of maintaining fluid and electrolyte levels, crucial for those managing potassium intake. This section provided invaluable insights into the symbiotic relationship between hydration, electrolyte balance, and dietary health, offering practical advice for integrating these elements into daily life.

Perhaps the most resonant chapters were those dedicated to "Mental and Emotional Well-being," where the narrative shifted to the psychological and emotional dimensions of dietary management. Through discussions on "Coping with Dietary Restrictions," "Seeking Support for Dietary Changes," and "Mindfulness and Stress Management Techniques," the book addressed the often-overlooked emotional challenges of navigating dietary restrictions. These sections offered a compassionate guide to finding balance and support in the face of dietary changes, reminding readers of the profound connection between mental health and physical well-being.

As we conclude this journey, it's clear that managing a low potassium diet is an intricate dance of nutrition, physical activity, mental resilience, and emotional support. This book has not only provided a roadmap for navigating the complexities of dietary management but also illuminated the path with empathy, understanding, and practical wisdom.

In closing, let us reflect on the words of Hippocrates, "Let food be thy medicine and medicine be thy food," a reminder that our journey to health transcends the physical. It's a holistic endeavor that nourishes the body, soothes the mind, and uplifts the spirit. May this book serve as a steadfast companion on your journey to wellness, inspiring you to embrace the richness of a balanced life, where every meal, every step, and every breath brings you closer to your healthiest self.